NATURAL HOMEMADE SKINCARE RECIPES

Must-Have DIY Skin Care Recipes for Glowing and Healthy Skin

Clair Simeon

TABLE OF CONTENT

TABLE OF CONTENTS

CHAPTER 1

Introduction - The Benefits of Natural and Organic Skincare

Recent years have seen a rise in the popularity of skincare products that use all-natural and organic components. Natural and organic skincare products are safer, healthier, and more environmentally friendly than their synthetically-based counterparts found in many popular brands.

Natural and organic skincare products have a lower potential to irritate the skin than their synthetic counterparts. Common side effects of using products with synthetic components include dryness, redness, and flaking. On the other hand, the natural and organic substances are frequently more mild and nourishing, making them appropriate for even the most delicate skin.

Natural and organic skincare products have no artificial ingredients or preservatives, which is another perk. Parabens, sulfates, and phthalates are common in commercial skincare products, and they have been linked to health problems like cancer and hormonal abnormalities. You can keep your skin safe from toxic chemicals by sticking to natural and organic products.

Natural and organic skincare products aren't just better for your skin since they don't contain harmful chemicals, but they can also improve your skin's health and beauty. Essential oils, plant extracts, and botanical oils are just a few examples of natural components that are packed with nourishing nutrients and antioxidants that can benefit the skin.

Using natural and organic skincare products can have positive effects on the environment in addition to the aforementioned advantages. The commercial skincare industry relies heavily on synthetic components, many of which are generated from non-renewable resources and hence have the potential to negatively influence the environment both during manufacturing and disposal. However, natural and organic products tend to be more eco-friendly because they use fewer synthetic additives and are derived from renewable resources. Your own carbon footprint can be reduced and you can help the beauty industry as a whole become more sustainable if you opt for natural and organic skincare products.

One further perk of organic and natural skin care products is that they typically smell better. Essential oils and other natural fragrances offer a more mild, natural perfume than the strong synthetic aromas utilized in many commercial skincare products.

The use of organic and natural skincare products is another way to take a more rounded approach to self-care. You can achieve inner and outer balance and harmony in your self-care activities by using skincare products made with natural ingredients.

In conclusion, there are many positive outcomes for your skin, your health, and the environment when you switch to organic and natural skincare products. What follows is an in-depth look at organic and natural skincare options, along with DIY formulas and instructions.

CHAPTER 2

Choosing the Right Ingredients for Your Skin Type

Using the appropriate components is essential when making your own organic and natural skin care products at home. It is crucial to choose substances that are appropriate for your skin type because they each have their own unique qualities and advantages.

Look for substances that control oil production and minimize inflammation if you have oily or acne-prone skin. Tea tree oil, witch hazel, and aloe vera are a few solid choices.

Look for elements that nourish and moisturize the skin if you have dry or sensitive skin. Avocado oil, shea butter, and coconut oil are all excellent choices.

Look for components that help to boost collagen production and skin suppleness if you have old or aging skin. Peptides that stimulate collagen production, vitamin C, and retinol are all viable choices.

You should take into account both your skin type and any particular skin concerns when choosing components. For under-eye bags and puffiness, for instance, substances like caffeine and Arnica can reduce inflammation and boost circulation, which can help alleviate your symptoms. Look for substances like licorice root or niacinamide, which help lighten and brighten the complexion, if you suffer from hyperpigmentation or an uneven skin tone.

In general, while selecting ingredients for your skincare products, it is most important to take into account your skin type and any specific concerns you may have. Based on these factors, we'll prescribe particular ingredients and provide recipes for various skincare products in the next chapters.

CHAPTER 3

Facial Cleansers and Toners: Natural Recipes for a Deep Clean

Remove grime, oil, and makeup as well as restore the skin's natural pH by following a skincare program that includes cleansing and toning. Natural and organic face cleansers and toners are discussed in this chapter, along with DIY recipes.

When it comes to facial cleansers, you may pick from a wide variety of all-natural and organic formulations. Here are a few things to keep an eye out for:

- Coconut oil is a natural, mild cleanser that does double duty as a skin-nourishing moisturizer and a powerful makeup remover.

- Olive oil and other plant oils are used to create Castile soap, a natural, plant-based soap. It cleanses well without drying out the skin and is very mild overall.

- Aloe vera is a natural substance that is both gentle and effective in terms of keeping the skin clean and hydrated.

- Oily or acne-prone skin can benefit from tea tree oil since it has antimicrobial ingredients that destroy bacteria and reduce irritation.

Make your own all-natural face cleanser with this easy recipe:
Ingredients:

- The equivalent of a quarter cup of coconut oil

- A Castile Soap Dish, 14 Cup

- a quarter cup of aloe vera gel

- 10 dilutions of tea tree oil

Instructions:

- In a small saucepan, melt the coconut oil over low heat.

- Turn off the heat and add the castile soap and aloe vera gel, mixing well.

- Add the tea tree oil and mix well.

- Store the finished product in the bathroom by pouring it into an airtight container.

- Use the cleanser by massaging a tiny quantity into your damp skin and then rinsing well with water.

Facial toners are used to restore the skin's natural pH balance and eliminate any lingering pollutants. Look for these organic and natural elements in a face toner:

- Rosewater, a natural skin toner, is known for its calming and hydrating effects.

- Apple cider vinegar is an all-natural toner that can be used to relieve inflammation and maintain the skin's natural pH.

- Witch hazel is an anti-inflammatory and anti-swelling natural toner.

- A natural toner, aloe vera calms and hydrates the skin.

This is a quick and easy face toner recipe:

Ingredients:

1/2 tsp. rosé

2 teaspoons of unfiltered apple cider vinegar

Witch hazel, 2 tbsp

Aloe vera gel, 2 teaspoons

Instructions:

Combine the aloe vera gel, witch hazel, apple cider vinegar, and rosewater in a small basin.

Store the finished product in the bathroom by pouring it into an airtight container.

After washing your face, add toner to a cotton pad and wipe your face with it. After that, apply some moisturizer.

CHAPTER 4

Moisturizers: Hydrating and Nourishing Recipes for All Skin Types

Because of their vital role in keeping the skin supple and healthy, moisturizers should never be skipped. Here we will discuss organic and all-natural moisturizers and give you recipes to make your own.

Moisturizers can contain a wide variety of natural and organic components; the ones that work best for your skin, however, will vary from person to person. Some of the things you'll need are:

Coconut oil is a wonderful natural moisturizer for all skin types, but especially dry and sensitive skin.

All skin types, especially dry or aged skin, can benefit from shea butter, as it is a natural, nutritious component.

Almond oil is a natural, lightweight oil that benefits oily and acne-prone skin the most.

Jojoba oil is a natural, lightweight oil that benefits oily or acne-prone skin the most.

Avocado oil is an all-natural moisturizer that is especially beneficial for dry or older skin.

For a natural moisturizer that works on all skin types, try this easy recipe:

Ingredients:

A Quarter Cup of Coconut Oil
Shea butter, about 2 tablespoons
Almond oil, 2 tablespoons
Amount: 2 tbsp. jojoba oil
Avocado oil, 1 tbsp

Instructions:

Combine the shea butter and coconut oil in a small saucepan and melt over low heat.

Put the pan on a cool surface and add the oils while stirring constantly.

Store the finished product in the bathroom by pouring it into an airtight container.

Use a pea-sized dollop of the moisturizer and massage it into your face and neck until it disappears.

Keep in mind that heavier oils like coconut oil and avocado oil can clog pores and exacerbate oily or acne-prone skin, so opt for something like almond oil or jojoba oil instead. Coconut oil and avocado oil are two thicker oils that may be better suited for dry or older skin than almond oil and jojoba oil. Try out various oils until you find one that works well with your skin.Recipes for Moisturizers that Hydrate and Nourish All Skin Types is Chapter 4

Because of their vital role in keeping the skin supple and healthy, moisturizers should never be skipped. Here we will discuss organic and all-natural moisturizers and give you recipes to make your own.

Moisturizers can contain a wide variety of natural and organic components; the ones that work best for your skin, however, will vary from person to person. Some of the things you'll need are:

Coconut oil is a wonderful natural moisturizer for all skin

types, but especially dry and sensitive skin.

All skin types, especially dry or aged skin, can benefit from shea butter, as it is a natural, nutritious component.

Almond oil is a natural, lightweight oil that benefits oily and acne-prone skin the most.

Jojoba oil is a natural, lightweight oil that benefits oily or acne-prone skin the most.

Avocado oil is an all-natural moisturizer that is especially beneficial for dry or older skin.

For a natural moisturizer that works on all skin types, try this easy recipe:

Ingredients:
A Quarter Cup of Coconut Oil
Shea butter, about 2 tablespoons
Almond oil, 2 tablespoons
Amount: 2 tbsp. jojoba oil
Avocado oil, 1 tbsp

Instructions:

Combine the shea butter and coconut oil in a small saucepan and melt over low heat.

Put the pan on a cool surface and add the oils while stirring constantly.

Store the finished product in the bathroom by pouring it into an airtight container.

Use a pea-sized dollop of the moisturizer and massage it into your face and neck until it disappears.

Keep in mind that heavier oils like coconut oil and avocado oil can clog pores and exacerbate oily or acne-prone skin, so opt for something like almond oil or jojoba oil instead. Coconut oil and avocado oil are two thicker oils that may be better suited for dry or older skin than almond oil and jojoba oil. Try out a few different oils until you find one that agrees with your skin.

CHAPTER 5

Exfoliators: Gentle and Effective Scrubs for Smooth, Radiant Skin

In order to get the smoothest, healthiest, and most radiant skin possible, exfoliators should be a regular part of your skincare routine. In this section, you'll learn about the benefits of exfoliators and how to make your own using all-natural ingredients.

Chemical exfoliators, such as alpha hydroxy acids (AHAs) and beta hydroxy acids (BHAs), dissolve dead skin cells, whereas physical exfoliators use abrasive particles to scrub them away.

Some common organic and natural components of physical exfoliants include:

Sugar is an excellent natural exfoliator since it is both mild and efficient.

When it comes to scrubbing away dead skin and clearing out pores, nothing beats salt, a natural exfoliator that's only a tad more abrasive than sugar.

Oatmeal is an excellent natural exfoliator because it is mild and nutritious, making it suitable for even the most delicate skin.

Natural exfoliants like ground nuts or seeds are ideal for sloughing off dead skin and opening up pores because of their mild abrasiveness.

Here's how to make a physical exfoliator from all-natural ingredients:

Ingredients:

Sugar, 1/2 cup

The equivalent of a quarter cup of coconut oil

10 optional drops of essential oil

To make this, combine the sugar and coconut oil in a separate bowl.
Blend in the aromatic oil if using.
Store the finished product in the bathroom by pouring it into an airtight container.
The exfoliant is applied in small amounts and massaged into damp skin in circular strokes.
Do a quick water rinse.

Those with more delicate skin should avoid using harsh exfoliants like sugar or salt and instead go for something like oatmeal or ground nuts and seeds.

Some examples of organic and natural substances that can be utilized in chemical exfoliants are listed below.

Glycolic acid, lactic acid, and citric acid are all examples of alpha hydroxy acids (AHAs), a class of naturally occurring exfoliants. In addition to reducing the appearance of fine wrinkles and uneven skin tone, AHAs are also effective at dissolving dead skin cells.

Beta hydroxy acid (BHA) is a naturally occurring exfoliant that helps remove dead skin cells and reduce inflammation. Salicylic acid is the most prevalent kind of BHA.

Papaya enzymes are a natural exfoliator that can be used to

get rid of dead skin and even out skin tone.

Make use of this easy chemical exfoliant recipe:

Ingredients:

2% Glycolic Acid 2 Tablespoons Aloe vera gel, 2 tablespoons 10 drops (optional) essential oil

Directions: Combine the glycolic acid and aloe vera gel in a small basin and set aside.

Blend in the aromatic oil if using.

Store the finished product in the bathroom by pouring it into an airtight container.

A small amount of the exfoliant should be massaged into your dry, clean skin in circular strokes. After that, apply some moisturizer.

It's crucial to remember that chemical exfoliants can be more powerful than physical ones, so it's best to start with a weaker dose and build up as necessary. Papaya enzymes are a milder exfoliant than alpha hydroxy acids (AHAs) and beta hydroxy acids (BHAs), and may be preferable for those with sensitive skin. Chemical exfoliants can make skin more sensitive to the sun, so protecting it with a broad-spectrum sunscreen is essential.

In general, exfoliators are a vital part of any skincare routine because they sweep away dulling dead skin cells and open up congested pores. Making your own natural and organic exfoliant at home can be a fun and inexpensive way to add exfoliation to your beauty routine, regardless of whether you prefer physical or chemical exfoliators.

CHAPTER 6

Face Masks: Nourishing Treatments for a Glowing Complexion

The addition of a face mask to your skincare routine is not only a treat for your face, but also an investment in its health. In this section, we'll discuss organic and all-natural ingredients that can be used to make your own facial masks.

distinct face masks have distinct purposes and advantages. Some common organic and natural face mask ingredients are as follows:

Masks made of clay are excellent in removing dirt and oil from the skin and restoring its natural balance. Bentonite clay and kaolin clay are two examples of useful natural clays.

Masks that add moisture and nourishment to the skin are

called hydrating masks. Honey, aloe vera, and avocados are some examples of beneficial all-natural products.

Masks that brighten the skin are helpful for reducing the look of dullness and blemishes. Lemon juice, papaya, and turmeric are all great all-natural options.

Calming and anti-inflammatory masks are what we mean when we talk about soothing masks. Chamomile, aloe vera, and green tea are some examples of helpful natural compounds.

The following is a straightforward clay face mask recipe:

Ingredients:

One-fourth cup of bentonite
14 cup of liquid
1.5 grams of honey
Optional: 10 drops of essential oil.

The bentonite clay, water, and honey should all be combined in a little bowl.

Add the essential oil to the mixture if using.

Avoid getting the mask in your eyes or mouth and apply it evenly to your face.

After 10 to 15 minutes, remove the mask and wash your face thoroughly.

In case your face might need some more moisture, try this easy homemade mask:

Ingredients:

14 cup of aloe vera gel

1-fourth of a cup of honey

Half of an avocado

1/25th of an olive

Instructions:

Blend the aloe vera gel and avocado together in a small bowl.

Add the honey and olive oil and mix well.

Avoid getting the mask in your eyes or mouth and apply it evenly to your face.

After 10 to 15 minutes, remove the mask and wash your face thoroughly.

Try this easy facial mask recipe for some natural radiance:

One-fourth cup of crushed papaya

1/4 cup water 1 tbsp. lemon juice

1.5 grams of honey

A Half Measure of Turmeric

Instructions:

Papaya, lemon juice, honey, and turmeric should be combined in a small bowl.

Avoid getting the mask in your eyes or mouth and apply it evenly to your face.

After 10 to 15 minutes, remove the mask and wash your face thoroughly.

In case your face might need some natural TLC, try this easy mask recipe:

Green tea, steeped and chilled to 1/4 cup

14 cup of aloe vera gel

Brew and cool 1 tablespoon of chamomile tea.

1.5 grams of honey

Instructions:

Green tea, aloe vera gel, chamomile tea, and honey should be combined in a small basin and stirred.

Avoid getting the mask in your eyes or mouth and apply it evenly to your face.

After 10 to 15 minutes, remove the mask and wash your face thoroughly.

In general, face masks are a wonderful way to replenish the skin, and there are many organic and natural varieties available. There is a natural face mask recipe for every skin care requirement, be it to remove excess oil, hydrate and moisturize, brighten and even out skin tone, or soothe and calm inflammation. An enjoyable and luxurious addition to any beauty routine is the use of face masks.

CHAPTER 8

Lip Balms: Moisturizing and Nourishing Recipes for Soft, Supple Lips

Lip balms are an integral element of any beauty routine because of its ability to hydrate and nourish the lips, preventing them from becoming dry and chapped. This section will discuss organic and all-natural lip balms, as well as provide recipes for making your own.

The finest lip balm for you will have ingredients tailored to your unique needs and skin type from among the many organic and natural options available. Some of the things you'll need are:

Beeswax is an all-natural substance that acts as a protective layer on the skin, keeping moisture in and toxins out.

Shea butter is an all-natural substance that is highly beneficial for dry and aged skin.

Coconut oil is a wonderful natural moisturizer for all skin types, but especially dry and sensitive skin.

Almond oil is a natural, lightweight oil that benefits

oily and acne-prone skin in particular.

Jojoba oil is a natural, lightweight oil that benefits oily or acne-prone skin the most.

Make your own all-natural lip balm with this easy recipe:

Ingredients:
Two tablespoons of shea butter One tablespoon of beeswax

1.25 grams of coconut oil

Almond oil, 1 tablespoon

Jojoba oil, one teaspoon

Instructions:

In a small saucepan, melt the shea butter, coconut oil, and beeswax together over low heat.

Turn off the stove and add the jojoba and almond oils, mixing well.

When the mixture has cooled and solidified, transfer it to an empty lip balm tube or tin.

A small amount of lip balm can be applied to the lips as needed.

Consider using a lip balm with fewer active ingredients if your skin is particularly sensitive. You can alter the formula to your liking by substituting oils or adding essential oils for fragrance.

In general, lip balms are an important element of any beauty routine because of how they help to nourish and hydrate the lips, making them more pliable and less dry. Making your own lip balm at home is a fun and inexpensive way to add this phase to your skincare routine, and there are many natural and organic products from which to select. There is a natural lip balm recipe for everyone, whether you choose a thicker balm or a thinner mixture.

CHAPTER 9

Hair Masks: Nourishing and Revitalizing Recipes for Healthy, Shiny Hair

Hair masks are a luxurious and nourishing supplement to your regular hair care routine that can help revive and restore dry, damaged hair. The alternatives for organic and natural hair masks, as well as instructions for making your own, will be discussed in this chapter.

There is a wide variety of hair masks available, and they all serve distinct purposes. The following are some examples of organic and natural components that can be utilized in various hair masks:

Egg yolks are rich in protein and other nutrients that are beneficial to hair health.

Honey is rich in antioxidants and is a great natural component for keeping hair healthy and hydrated.

Olive oil is rich in fatty acids and is a great natural ingredient for nourishing and moisturizing dry, damaged hair.

Avocado is rich in fatty acids and is a great natural

ingredient for nourishing and moisturizing hair.

Coconut milk is rich in fatty acids and can be used to both nourish and hydrate the hair.

A natural protein hair mask can be made with the following ingredients.

Ingredients:

Two whole eggs
1.5 grams of honey

1/4 cup water 1 tbsp olive oil

The recipe calls for combining the egg yolks, honey, and olive oil in a small bowl.

The second step is to apply the concoction to freshly washed hair, beginning at the roots and working your way out.

Leave the mask on for 20 to 30 minutes, preferably with a shower cap or plastic wrap covering your hair.

Warm water should be used to remove the mask, and your regular shampoo and conditioner should be used afterward.

In case your hair might need some more moisture, try this easy mask recipe:

One-half of an avocado, mashed

Milk from 1/4 of a coconut

1.5 grams of honey

Instructions: Mash   the avocado with the coconut milk and honey in a small bowl until smooth.

Working from the roots to the ends, apply the mixture to freshly washed hair.

Leave the mask on for 20 to 30 minutes, preferably with a shower cap or plastic wrap covering your hair.

Warm water should be used to remove the mask, and your regular   shampoo   and conditioner should be used afterward.

In general, hair masks are a luxurious and nourishing complement to your regular hair care routine, helping to revive and restore damaged or dull hair. There are a wide variety of natural and organic substances available, including protein for strengthening the hair and fatty acids for moisturizing and nourishing the hair. Hair masks are a fun and luxurious addition to any hair care routine, allowing you to pamper your hair while pampering yourself. If you want clean, well-maintained hair, use your regular shampoo and conditioner afterward.

CHAPTER 10

Body Scrubs: Exfoliating and Nourishing Recipes for Smooth, Radiant Skin

Scrubbing the entire body is a crucial part of any beauty routine since it helps get rid of dulling dead skin and opens up blocked pores. This chapter delves into the world of organic and all-natural body scrubs, along with DIY instructions.

Scrubbing your body can be done in many different ways, each with its own set of advantages. Some examples of organic and natural substances that can be utilized in body scrubs are listed below.

Sugar is an excellent exfoliant because it is both natural and mild.

For rougher, thicker skin, try an exfoliant like salt, which is all-natural and more abrasive.

Coffee is an excellent exfoliant since it is both natural and stimulating, helping to boost circulation and diminish the appearance of cellulite.

Oats are a wonderful exfoliant because they are mild and safe even for the most delicate skin.

Baking soda is an excellent natural exfoliant that also helps maintain a healthy skin pH and reduce irritation.

A sugar body scrub can be made at home with this easy recipe:

Ingredients:

1 mug of sugar
1,25 ounces of almond oil

10 optional drops of essential oil

Instructions:

Combine the sugar and almond oil in a separate bowl.

Blend in the aromatic oil if using.

Store the finished product in the bathroom by pouring it into an airtight container.

Scrub a little quantity into damp skin and massage in a circular motion to apply.

Please use water to wash off.

Here's how to make a salt scrub at home:

Ingredients:

1 pound salt

Two-thirds of a cup of olive oil

10 optional drops of essential oil

The salt and olive oil should be combined in a little bowl.

Blend in the aromatic oil if using.

Store the finished product in the bathroom by pouring it into an airtight container.

Scrub a little quantity into damp skin and massage in a circular motion to apply. Please use water to wash off.

In general, using a body scrub is a great way to improve the appearance of your skin by sloughing off dead cells and dirt that has accumulated in your pores. Many different types of natural and organic materials can be used as exfoliators, from sugar and oats to salt and coffee. It can be both enjoyable and cost-effective to make your own body scrub at home and use it as part of your regular skincare routine. To get the best results, use an exfoliator designed for your skin type and address any remaining issues with a hydrating moisturizer.

CHAPTER 11

Foot Soaks: Relaxing and Revitalizing Recipes for Tired, Achy Feet

Soothing tired, aching feet and boosting general wellness, foot soaks are a wonderful addition to any self-care routine. In this section, you'll learn about organic and all-natural ingredients that can be used to make your own foot soaks at home.

Numerous kinds of foot soaks exist, each with its own special advantages. The following are some examples of organic and natural materials that can be utilized in various foot soaks:

Epsom salts are rich in magnesium and can be used to treat a variety of ailments, including edema, poor circulation, and tense muscles.

Baking soda is a natural
substance that helps maintain
a healthy pH level and lessen
inflammation.

Essential lavender oil is a
wonderful stress reliever and
calming agent.

The anti-inflammatory and
antibacterial properties of tea
tree oil are well-documented.

Ginger is a natural remedy that helps increase blood flow and decrease swelling.

Formula for an all-natural Epsom salt foot soak:

Ingredients:

Epsom salts, one cup
Essential oil of lavender, 10 drops
A warm pint of water

Instructions:

Combine the Epsom salts and lavender oil in a small bowl.

Warm the water and add it to the ingredients in a large basin or foot tub.

After 20 to 30 minutes, drain the solution and wash your feet.

A natural baking soda foot soak can be made using this easy recipe:

Half a cup of baking soda
Tea tree oil, 10 drops

A warm pint of water

Instructions:

Add the tea tree oil to the baking soda in a small bowl and stir to combine.

Warm the water and add it to the ingredients in a large basin or foot tub.

3. Soak your feet for 20 to 30 minutes in the solution, and then wash them off with water.

Soaking your feet is a great way to unwind after a long day, relieve foot pain, and boost your health and wellness. Epsom salts are great for reducing swelling and improving circulation, baking soda is great for balancing pH and reducing inflammation, lavender essential oil is great for relieving stress, and tea tree oil is great for fighting bacteria and reducing inflammation. Add a foot bath to your self-care routine for a luxurious and easy way to pamper your feet. You should pick an item that will address your specific problems, and then use a moisturizer to keep your skin healthy and protected.